Laure Goldbright

I0123300

Menopause Free of Suffering:

A Testimonial

Menopause is Not a Disease! Hot flashes,
Low Mood, Weight gains, and Other
Menopausal Symptoms Can Be Avoided

Buenos Books America
www.buenosbooks.us

©Laure Goldbright - 2022
http://lauregoldbright.buenosbooks.fr

ISBN: 978-1-963580-03-7
Imprint: Buenos Books America
www.buenosbooks.us

INTRODUCTION: Menopause is wrongly accused of everything!

In her fifties, my friend Annie began suffering from annoying spells of dizziness. Since she no longer had her periods, she naturally attributed this problem to menopause, and her doctor was in complete agreement. Therefore, she began taking drugs to "fight the menopause," which unfortunately had no effect on her dizziness at all. The disorder was ruining her life and causing increasing anxiety and sadness. Everything she tried (drugs, herbal teas, psychotherapy, etc.) had no effect and she was desperate.

Fortunately, after some time, having resigned herself to living with her "menopausal disability," she was lucky enough to accidentally break her glasses and forced to consult an ophthalmologist, who prescribed new glasses better suited to her sight. With these new glasses, Annie was pleasantly surprised to notice that her dizziness had gone! So her troubles had simply been caused by her old glasses, which over time had become ill-adapted to her sight! However, as she was in her fifties, no one, not even she herself, had thought of looking for the actual cause instead of automatically attributing it to menopause.

Annie's case is just one among many that demonstrates just how common damaging ideas about menopause are! From a certain age, when a woman is unwell, we automatically attribute it to menopause and no longer try to understand what is happening in her body and what could be done naturally to regain perfect health. This common Western belief that from the onset of menopause women "fall apart" is incredible. If it is true that in nature everything is born, evolves, ages, and dies, there is no reason to accept that from the middle of her life a woman should "collapse" due to a simple and natural hormonal change. On the contrary, some women have found this life stage to be a positive and tranquil experience. I am one of them, but it didn't happen by chance.

In my family, women have tended to face a lot of ailments before, during, and after menopause. As I had no wish to suffer like them, I decided to take action. I challenged all our Western beliefs about menopause and did some research to find out what I could do to avoid related issues. I was determined to experience a happy menopause without hot flashes, low mood, insomnia, nervousness, depression, accumulation of cellulite, dark spots on the face, and accelerated aging. And I achieved it!

I realized that almost all the disorders culturally attributed to menopause are actually due to other causes, which can be eliminated. In this book, I will share with you the keys I have discovered to a serene, joyful, peaceful, and natural menopause, despite my family's hereditary background. I will let you in on my methods of investigation and then share some important advice so that you too, can avoid so-called "menopausal symptoms." Even if you are already suffering from a menopausal symptom, it is not too late to take action and regain well-being naturally.

This small book, easy to read and free of medical jargon, will help you stay fit, healthy, happy, and beautiful despite menopause. You will see and understand for yourself the actual causes of almost all the ailments mistakenly attributed to menopause. You will then learn how to avoid them without medication and without spending a fortune.

CHAPTER 1: The actual causes of almost all the disorders mistakenly attributed to menopause

When the women in my family go through menopause, they gain weight or become skinny, and suffer from terrible menopause symptoms. I have seen the whole "clinical picture" of every conceivable menopausal symptom in my mother, my three older sisters, and my aunts.

I was only in my thirties when my mother started programming me to suffer this "hereditary martyrdom." "You will see," she admonished me quite theatrically and with a gloomy face, "this blood that no longer goes out from below rises to our heads and poisons us." I thought that she was totally irrational, and inside myself I laughed at her strange opinion. But, later on, I understood that she had a good perception of her body and was partly right.

Despite my mother always complaining and telling us all the details of her menopausal symptoms, I intuitively felt deep inside that menopause could be experienced otherwise, and that all these ailments were avoidable. I started asking myself some questions and trying to understand why, in our modern Western society, almost all women suffer from menopausal symptoms long before, during, and after menopause. It is true that mainstream media and the pharmaceutical industry program us to believe that menopause is a kind of disease - almost a disability - that affects women "who have passed their sell date." Fortunately, despite all this propaganda, some women live this life stage in peace and good health, although the mainstream media avoids speaking about them.

Here are the main questions I asked myself before doing my personal research:

- Why should women's bodies suddenly "collapse" due to a natural hormonal change, while they have experienced changes without problems?

- Girls are not sick before puberty. Why should women be sick after their last periods?

- What happens during menstruation that is so important to a woman's health, and stops with menopause?

- Why do so many women complain of so many menopausal symptoms, and why do some women have no problems?

- Why do almost all the women in my family experience menopause in such a terrible way, and what can I do to avoid this sad fate?

I have never had a research laboratory or research funds available to me. But I think I had something much better: good communication with my body and the presence of my mother and three older sisters, who I have observed closely for many years To understand what was happening to the menopausal women in my family, I thought it was important to observe their appearance and behavior before, during, and after their periods, when they still had them, and then during their menopause. My personal research allowed me to understand how it is possible to experience a happy menopause, without hot flashes, low mood, insomnia, nervousness, depression, accumulation of cellulite, dark spots around the eyes, age spots, and accelerated aging.

For now, I am the only exception to the terrible way women in my family have always experienced menopause. Unfortunately, my younger sisters did not followed my advice and did not escape the usual family fate. Often nothing can be done for our closest relatives. It annoys a lot of the tribe's members if one of them challenges their deep-rooted habits. Fortunately, I can now share this with many other people. With this testimonial, I hope to help you avoid almost all the symptoms commonly attributed to menopause and positively consider this stage of your life. The more women understand how their bodies work, how to live well through menopause, and how to take advantage of it, the more we will change the negative image of menopausal women, imposed on them for many centuries by our civilization. I hope that many older women will become examples for younger women, so they will no longer dread their future. They will see through their example that menopause is not a disease at all. It is truly a natural and positive transformation for a normal woman. If menopause is lived well and not hindered, the energetic change it triggers frees the energy of women from the natural purpose of procreation toward other interesting purposes. With such examples of successful transformations, younger women will not be worried or panicked when they also approach menopause. Some may even be in a hurry to get there, for the wonderful feeling of freedom that well-lived menopause can bring.

11

When I was in my twenties, a friend of mine in her forties, who was probably very afraid of menopause, used to make fun of women in their fifties and called them "menopausal grannies." (In French the phrase sounds ridiculous and funny: "mémé ménopausée"!) I was shocked by her attitude. Later, I understood that she had only stored and then transmitted the negative image of femininity that deeply permeates our patriarchal society. Comedians, even female ones, do not hesitate to make people laugh at the expense of menopausal women. This is bad. Women deserve respect as human beings, regardless of their age and fertility potential. I hope that my testimonial will encourage other women to act, so that together we can contribute to changing these disastrous stereotypes about menopausal women. Women naturally have other powers besides those related to sex, seduction, or procreation. Such powers have always existed, but our modern, materialistic world obviously does not want to hear about them, and many women ignore their existence. In ancient times the existence of such powers was accepted, but not always welcome, especially by the Church.

When they reach menopause and after they figure out how to stay fit and healthy, women's spiritual faculties can develop more easily than in most men. If not hindered, all the energy that is no longer used for menstruation, procreation, and often also sex, automatically goes up to the spiritual centers of the brain and activates them. This seems a little more difficult for men. This is probably why yogis have devised so many practices and exercises for the ascent of kundalini (energy located in the lower body) to the higher centers. Furthermore, by nature and social conditioning, men tend to have their energy trapped "in the lower part of their bodies" - for sex and procreation - up to a very advanced age, and sometimes with the help of modern medical "crutches."

Women can take advantage of menopause to considerably increase their personal power, energy, and creativity and be happier and vibrant. Many women are not aware of these possibilities and have no idea of the beautiful horizon that can open up for them with menopause. It is much better than the depressing devaluation that society imposes on our minds.

Negative ideas and fears decrease the energy level in the body. And a low energy level is not conducive to the emergence of these new abilities in women. If traditional Chinese medicine says that menopause is "the second spring of women," it is because at this time women can renew their energy and use it for other purposes. True, "creation through the lower part of the body" comes to an end, but all the energy that was directed to the lower centers of the body is now available for the "higher centers" of the brain and for other kinds of "creations" (spiritual, artistic, intellectual) and capacities considered paranormal.

If they want and if they find a suitable partner, menopausal women can also experience emotional and human exchanges of a higher spiritual level. With menopause, sexual energy goes to the top of the body and powerfully activates a woman's brain and "heart" powers. The desire and will to create become stronger and their "words" are more powerful.

I was lucky enough to understand in time that almost all ailments attributed to menopause are not normal, do not result from menopause, and are perfectly preventable.

Despite the progress of medical knowledge and techniques, there is still a lot to discover about the functioning of the human body. Not to mention, our physical health also strongly depends on our way of thinking. Sometimes it is enough to believe in the virtues of a remedy or a placebo to immediately feel better.

In contrast, the widespread and disastrous ideas about menopause have a *nocebo* effect, making women believe they must get chronically ill and "collapse" by the age of fifty. Fortunately, these are just ideas (bad ones), and it is possible to replace them with good ones, bringing joy, well-being, good health, and serenity to menopausal women.

This is possible. It happened to me and it can also happen to you if you understand the true causes of so-called menopausal symptoms and follow three basic steps to avoid them.

I will not go into the details of "menopausal symptoms": hot flashes, night sweats, depression, sadness, irritability, vaginal dryness, accelerated aging, insomnia, urinary disorders, decreased blood pressure, low libido, mood, production of hormones, loss of bone density, gum infections, fluid retention, memory loss, cognitive deterioration, etc. Of course, not everything decreases with menopause - some increase: weight and belly fat, cellulite, cardiovascular risks, age spots, wrinkles, and dark circles around the eyes! In short, if we consider only common ideas and mainstream media publications, menopause can only be a nightmarish and inevitable perspective!

Science claims that menopausal symptoms are triggered by hormonal deficits due to the ovaries stopping their production; and mainstream medicine tries to remedy menopausal symptoms by compensating with hormones for the alleged deficit. As for the skin, weight, and appearance, they create joy for all the thriving "beauty and diet industries."

Let's object to the science that before puberty ovaries are not active; at that time girls are healthy and have no hot flashes or other menopausal symptoms! Alternatively, if we closely observe men, we will soon notice that they, too, suffer from hot flashes and night sweats from a certain age, especially if they have a big belly. They rarely complain about it, and their doctors naturally attribute this "decline" to other health conditions and not to andropause. Sometimes men start having hot flashes and night sweats in their forties and for the rest of their lives! The present book is intended mainly for women, but it can also help men who want to know how they can avoid so-called andropause symptoms.

For my part, I have observed that menopausal symptoms are not a result of hormonal changes in the body due to inactive ovaries. Such symptoms are caused by something else. By the way, did you notice that most of the time we do not talk about "hormonal changes," but we dramatize this situation using the expression the "hormonal disruption of menopause." While I was writing this book, I found medical confirmation of my observations in a book by American doctor Hulda Clark, who explained that when the ovaries stop their hormonal work, the adrenal glands take their turn to perform this task in the body.

Hulda Clark's book is entitled *The Cure for All Diseases*. Here are some interesting quotes:

"*Insomnia, irritability, PMS (premenstrual syndrome), depression, anxiety, nervousness, are all not to be expected at and after menopause. They may certainly be caused by hormone imbalances. It is these imbalances that are not normal. NO menopausal symptoms are normal.*"

And she continues: "*After the ovaries are done with their cycles of estrogen and progesterone* *production, the **adrenal glands'** hormone production was meant to "kick in" and make up any deficit."*

"At the end (of the fertile period) the adrenal glands can continue to maintain your hormonal balance."

She then explains why the adrenal glands are often prevented from maintaining hormonal balance. She claims that it is enough to rid the body of parasites and pollutants, to restore hormonal balance, and to make the hot flashes and other symptoms commonly attributed to menopause disappear as if with a magic wand.

How did I figure out that it is not the hormonal change due to the inactivation of the ovaries that causes so-called menopausal symptoms? It was mainly through observing what occurs during periods. The most important difference between menopausal women and others is not the inactivity of ovaries but the disappearance of menstruation. In my opinion, scientists have not yet sufficiently observed the phenomenon of menstruation. By observing what happens during her periods, every woman can understand the causes of most of the symptoms attributed to menopause and avoid them. I'll explain why.

Did you observe what happened inside you before, during, and after your periods? I have done it for years and have also observed the behavior and appearance of my older sisters when they still had their periods, as well as after. By the time they reached the age of menopause, the women in my family looked duller, less radiant, and less clean. They got sick more often, they tended to be more negative, more pessimistic, and more often in a bad mood. So far nothing new compared to popular beliefs about menopause. But for years I had been carefully observing what happened when we had our periods.

I could see that when my older sisters were about to have their periods, they seemed a little less lively, less clean, more irritable, and more tired. After their periods they looked fitter, renewed, and cleaned up. Pimples, dull skin, bad mood, and water retention were gone. In myself I observed that the main effect of menses was a cleansing of my body from the impurities accumulated due to the bad lifestyle I lived then. During my periods I sweated a lot, especially at night, and I was often too hot. My body was eliminating a lot of toxins, and I was helping this natural process by getting as much rest as possible and drinking warm water to encourage elimination. I knew from experience, and from my observations of other family members that colds, flu, unsightly pimples, and other ailments magically disappeared after our menses.

After my periods I always felt cleaner, lighter, and I had a sense of renewed energy flowing through my body. I was "deflated" and generally lost some fat, especially on my stomach. If my intestinal transit was blocked before my periods, it would return to normal with them, and sometimes I also had beneficial diarrhea. My skin was more beautiful and my good mood and zest for life were powerfully back. Periods always freed me from any negative states I had before: anger, ruminations, and dark thoughts went away with the toxins. If I had suffered from insomnia, irritability, stress, or anxiety before my periods, everything was fine after them. Serenity and normal sleep came back.

In scientific books there are many details on the role of hormones in the female cycle. Menstruation is explained by the fact that when an ovum has not been fertilized, the body no longer needs the endometrium, *i.e.,* the membrane that had formed to receive a fertilized ovum and eliminates it. According to science, it is the elimination of this membrane that gives rise to a woman's cycle. Scientific explanation of menstruation ends there. This seems correct, but incomplete. To understand what happens during menstruation, we need to go further, because women not only get rid of the endometrium during their periods, but also eliminate many other visible and invisible things. If you are a woman, you don't need to be a scientist or have a laboratory to do your own experiments, or to understand the other very important functions of menstruation not considered by mainstream science.

As long as she observes herself carefully, every woman can feel inside herself that, in addition to eliminating the endometrium, the most important function of menstruation is to cleanse the body of accumulated impurities and toxins, and to clear the mind of its own negativity. You can also take steps to support these natural processes, and amplify their good effects on your skin, weight, and health.

We live in a patriarchal civilization, where for millennia women have been considered inferior to men. But Nature has a different "opinion" of women. Women matter much more to Nature than men, because they play a much more important role in the perpetuation of the species and in the renewal of life. I personally believe that men and women are equal and that they complement each other. But to Nature a male is not as important as a female, because it would take only a few men to impregnate thousands of women. To put women in the best possible conditions to ensure the perpetuation of the species, Nature has endowed them with a great advantage, which she did not grant to men.

Contrary to appearances and common beliefs, menstruation is not an unnecessary annoyance affecting women; instead, it is the biggest advantage they have ever had over men. Thanks to menstruation, women regularly and automatically eliminate toxins for a large part of their life, and for this reason women have a longer life expectancy than men. This is despite the fact that pregnancy and giving birth take a toll on their bodies, and that they have to deal with the deplorable and disturbing image of femininity in patriarchal societies. To get pregnant, carry a baby for nine months, give birth without dying, then breastfeed babies and raise them, women need to be in good physical and psychological condition. Since a body full of toxins and obstructed by waste is not conducive to good health, Nature has devised an automatic and mandatory process, in tune with the great cosmic rhythms, so that every woman of childbearing age, whatever her social status, rich or poor, has their body and mind cleansed. This process occurs during their periods. Therapeutic bloodletting practiced in the past by doctors probably originated in an attempt to imitate the process of blood purification, naturally performed by menstruation.

Today we have widely forgotten that menses not only eliminates the endometrium when no fertilization takes place, but it also deeply purifies the body and mind to increase the odds of future pregnancy. In ancient civilizations, it was well known that women eliminated their toxins during their periods. For this reason they could not access temples or perform some activities during their periods because they were considered unclean, since it was known that this was the time when they were getting rid of their mind and body "garbage." Since men could enter sanctuaries without any restrictions, even when they had such an unhealthy lifestyle that they had become "walking garbage bins," I thought that putting women aside under this pretense was perhaps only a pretext to give them the opportunity to rest and purify themselves. Certain ancient people were closer than we are to Nature, and they knew better. They considered existence more wisely. Today, it would still do a lot of good for busy working women if they could rest during their periods.

The greater longevity of women compared to men is mainly due to the fact that, for about forty years of their lives, women are naturally constrained to an automatic and cyclical cleansing of their body. Men don't have this natural advantage. As a result, they generally have a much shorter lifespan than women. If men took action to regularly eliminate the toxins from a young age they would have a longer life expectancy.

When women are no longer of childbearing age, they are on par with men, at least in terms of toxins that accumulate in the body over time. As soon as menstruation slows down and becomes less effective in cleaning the body, women should take the necessary steps to help their body regularly eliminate toxins. Otherwise, they will quickly become overloaded by all the toxins they are no longer automatically eliminating each month. Such quick accumulation of "waste" in the body inevitably triggers the so-called menopausal symptoms that are actually caused by an important built up of toxins and deposits, hindering the proper functioning of the body.

PMS (premenstrual symptoms) affecting some younger women are also caused by an overload of toxins that the body cannot manage to eliminate even when the "automatic system" is still in operation. They give to women of childbearing age a glimpse of the future menopausal symptoms they can expect if they continue with the lifestyle that is causing the cluttering of their bodies.

Some women never suffer from PMS, because they have few toxins and waste to eliminate during their periods. Whenever young women have many ailments akin to "menopausal symptoms" during their periods, most of the time it is because their "cleaning system" is overwhelmed.

In summary, we can say that:

THE MOST IMPORTANT DIFFERENCE BETWEEN WOMEN OF REPRODUCTIVE AGE AND MENOPAUSAL WOMEN IS THAT THE FIRST REGULARLY ELIMINATE THEIR ACCUMULATED TOXINS VIA THEIR PERIODS, WHILE THE SECOND CONTINUE ACCUMULATING MORE AND MORE TOXINS IN THEIR BODIES.

MENOPAUSAL SYMPTOMS ARE NOT CAUSED BY THE END OF THE ACTIVITY OF THEIR OVARIES, BUT BY THE

GRADUAL INTOXICATION OF THEIR BODIES.

MEN WHO HAVE INTOXICATED BODIES ALSO SUFFER FROM SIMILAR SYMPTOMS, PARTICULARLY FROM HOT FLASHES AND NIGHT SWEATS.

SUCH AILMENTS BEGIN IN MEN AND WOMEN AS SOON AS THEIR BODIES ARE OVERLOADED WITH TOXINS.

THE ACTUAL CAUSE OF SO-CALLED MENOPAUSAL SYMPTOMS IS NOT HORMONAL CHANGES RESULTING FROM THE INACTIVITY OF OVARIES, BUT AN OVERLOAD OF TOXINS IN THE BODY HINDERING ITS CORRECT FUNCTIONING.

TOXINS IN THE BLOOD, COMPACT AND HARDENED FECES BLOCKED FOR YEARS IN THE INTESTINE, BILE STONES IN THE LIVER AND GALLBLADDER, MUD IN THE

BLADDER, AND MUCUS THROUGHOUT THE WHOLE BODY ALL HINDER THE NORMAL FUNCTIONING OF THE BODY AND CREATE SO-CALLED MENOPAUSAL SYMPTOMS.

THE SOLUTION TO AVOID "MENOPAUSAL SYMPTOMS" IS VERY SIMPLE: THEY CAN BE AVOIDED BY REGULARLY CLEANSING THE BODY.

Obviously, this is a cleansing of the inside of the body, because women today do a lot for the outside of their bodies. They wash themselves, put on make-up to hide the effects of body toxins on skin, and apply perfume to mask bad odor caused by toxins and deposits in the body. Instead of wasting so much time trying to mask all these symptoms, why not eliminate their root cause by regularly doing internal body cleansing?

The most problematic part of the body for the accumulation of waste is the digestive tract, especially the large and small intestines. Therefore, it is important to have good hygiene and to do intestinal cleansing regularly. Over the years deposits build up on the walls of the intestines, which progressively slows down their proper functioning. This leads to a poor metabolism and an increase in fermentation and putrefaction toxins, further amplified by the slowing down of the peristaltic movement and bowel movement. This is where the vicious circle usually begins, and if not controlled leads to "menopausal symptoms," then to premature senility, and to a shortened life expectancy.

As I wrote above, I finally understood that my mother was partly right when she said (in a way which seemed irrational to me at the time): "This blood that no longer comes out from below, goes up to our heads and poisons our lives."

She had very good communication with her body. Of course, toxin-laden blood does not circulate properly in the brain, and therefore it really poisons our body and our life, as she put it.

Despite the fact that all the women in my family had to suffer from terrible menopausal ailments, I can testify that thanks to the toxin elimination practices I have used, I completely avoided all their common "menopausal symptoms."

I could stop here, because the most important thing has been said, but it is important to speak about the three most effective techniques for eliminating and/or avoiding toxins. They have more or less fallen into oblivion and many women don't know them. Modern schools of medicine are now more focused on diseases and drugs than on natural internal cleansing techniques that help maintain good health. Yet these techniques have been used by men and women since the dawn of time: they consist of intestinal hygiene, fasting, and deworming. These are the most effective, but there are many other ways to help the body eliminate toxins, such as saunas, massages, baths, sports, castor oil poultices, clay poultices, thermal baths, etc.

In 2012 I published a small book on the benefits of colon cleansing[1] that I invite you to read for more details on this practice. In the present book I will briefly mention the intestinal hygiene techniques that are available to us, and I will talk about a device that I learned about after the publication of my book on colon cleansing.

Let's talk about the most effective ways to prevent so-called menopausal symptoms.

---

[1] *Colon Cleansing and its benefits for health and skin: Testimonial*, How I regained a flat stomach, slim waist, peaceful sleep, and healthy skin without age spots by cleansing my colon with colonic irrigation, Laure Goldbright.

CHAPTER 2: Two effective techniques for eliminating toxins and avoiding menopausal symptoms

Do you remember my observations on the most important processes that take place during periods?

- Increase in body temperature;

- Sweating and increased body odor;

- Elimination of toxins and sometimes phlegm through menstrual blood;

- Mood improvement;

- Relief of nervous tensions;

- Weight loss and elimination of water retention;

- Improvement of bowel movement.

Some techniques that man has used since the dawn of time to purify the body are mere imitations of the effects of menstruation or fever. I would like to say a few words about fever before returning to our topic. Fever is a process that raises the body temperature to dissolve and evacuate certain deposits and toxins. Our bodies are incredibly intelligent and often create "diseases" on their own to purify and cure themselves. Too bad we no longer listen to our bodies, and we even fight its beneficial mechanisms with drugs, thereby obstructing its elimination processes and forcing it to "shut up." Unfortunately, in this case, the day comes when we are forced to listen to the body constantly because of pain. When we reach old age with a body overwhelmed by the accumulated waste of a lifetime and all the parasites that can better strive in it, we cannot live without suffering. There are many practices that attest to the importance of raising body temperature to remove toxins. I think that hot flashes and night sweats are means, akin to fever, used by the body to promote the elimination of toxins. Many means have been invented to raise body temperature and induce sweating: the sweat huts of South American shamans, Nordic saunas, Oriental hammam, the sweat baths of the ancient Romans and Greeks, modern infrared saunas, and the baths of Doctor Salmanoff (very hot baths with Siberian larch essences, to unclog the capillaries and reactivate blood microcirculation), to name a few. Intense physical exercise also helps eliminate toxins by increasing body temperature. In traditional medicine attempts have been made to artificially induce "fever" so that the body can burn its toxins and heal itself. Instead, modern medicine almost always fights fever and tries to stop it with drugs.

Water also helps eliminate toxins from the body. "Drink and eliminate!" was the message of a French advertisement for a brand of mineral water. It first showed a tired and sad person, with a dull face. After drinking the excellent water, this person took off her dull and tired face as if it were a mask, revealing a smiling, radiant face, glowing with excellent health.

Water is a true gift of Nature; it promotes purification of body and mind. There are about a hundred spas in France whose waters help cure or better manage all kinds of pathologies. There are also many in Italy and other countries. Unfortunately, spa treatments are of little use to people with a clogged digestive tract.

Drinking water, even thermal water, is not enough to free the intestine from all the waste that has accumulated on its walls for many years, and has become so compacted and dry it is very difficult to get rid of.

There are different ways to use water to free the intestines from these deposits: enemas, modern machines for colonic irrigation, and other devices like "my perfect colon," which was invented by an Italian company. This is a smart and inexpensive device, costing only around 60 USD, that makes intestinal cleansing at home easy. It is simple to use, connecting to a sink or shower faucet. It is composed of a set of small, linked tubes, equipped with a manual system for controlling the flow of water; it ends with a cannula to be inserted into the rectum while sitting on the toilet.

The "My Perfect Colon" device can be used sitting on the toilet (there is a support with suction cups that can be attached to the toilet), or lying down on an enema board or an air mattress also manufactured by this innovative company. For my part, I only use part of the device, which I put in the photo below, because it is much more effective to use it squatting on the toilet rather than sitting in a position that is not conducive to emptying the colon. It is a great product, very light, efficient, affordable, and easy to use. Travel accessories are also available to connect this system almost anywhere.

If you also buy the enema board or enema air mattress (which are quite expensive), you will be able to clean the whole colon quietly at home. But the temperature of the tap water should be stable. If you want to use it effectively while sitting on the toilet, you will need enough water pressure. (Pressure that is too high is not a problem because the device has a valve for automatic control of water pressure). Good pressure is less important when lying down. Using longer cannulas would be more effective when lying down, but they don't sell them at present. You can easily use this device even if the toilet is far from a tap by simply connecting an extension pipe up to three meters long. This device is more practical and hygienic than enema bags. With regard to common enemas, the transparent tubes of most have grooves inside, and are therefore hard to clean. Bacteria accumulate there, and even mold. Instead, the inside of the pipes used in My Perfect Colon are smooth. The device comes with a small water filtering system.

Picture of the device "My Perfect Colon":

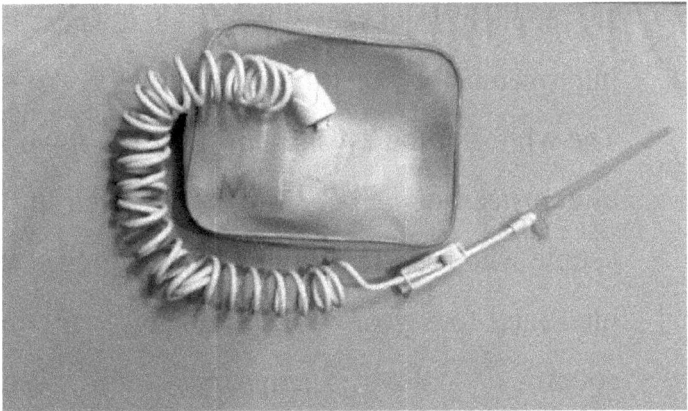

On *YouTube* there are many videos, especially in English, presenting do-it-yourself devices to clean the colon at home. Cleansing the colon at home is better than doing nothing; but the most effective way to deeply cleanse the colon is colonic irrigation performed by a trained therapist equipped with a good hydrotherapy machine, and who massages the belly or feet during the sessions. I describe in detail the professional machine for colon hydrotherapy in my book on intestinal hygiene. As far as I know, nothing more effective for colon cleansing has yet been invented. A few sessions and a preparatory diet are enough to achieve visible and spectacular improvement of health and, especially, the skin. The whites of the eyes return to a natural whitish-blue instead of being yellowish, as seen in most people who have been living with a clogged large intestine for years. Unfortunately, in many countries colonic irrigations are usually expensive and not reimbursed by health insurance because they are not medically approved. Wikipedia quotes a mainstream doctor: "The colon cleanses itself... The idea that its walls are coated with years-old hamburger residue is preposterous."[2]

Yet, thanks to technological advances it is now possible to swallow a tiny camera enclosed in a capsule and see fecal impactions and parasites in the digestive tract of some sick people. Some videos on "video capsules endoscopy" on *YouTube* have shown this evidence.

I have met many doctors in France who have never experienced colonic irrigation, seen one of these machines, nor observed the results of these irrigations on their patients. They claim that colonic irrigations are dangerous, and they frighten their patients whenever they want advice on this topic. Fortunately, there are more and more doctors who are open to other perspectives and accept looking at reality. A doctor friend, after noticing the good results of my first three

---

[2] https://en.wikipedia.org/wiki/Colon_cleansing

colonic irrigations, completely changed his mind and started having colonic cleansings and recommending them to his patients.

Picture of a professional colon irrigation machine:

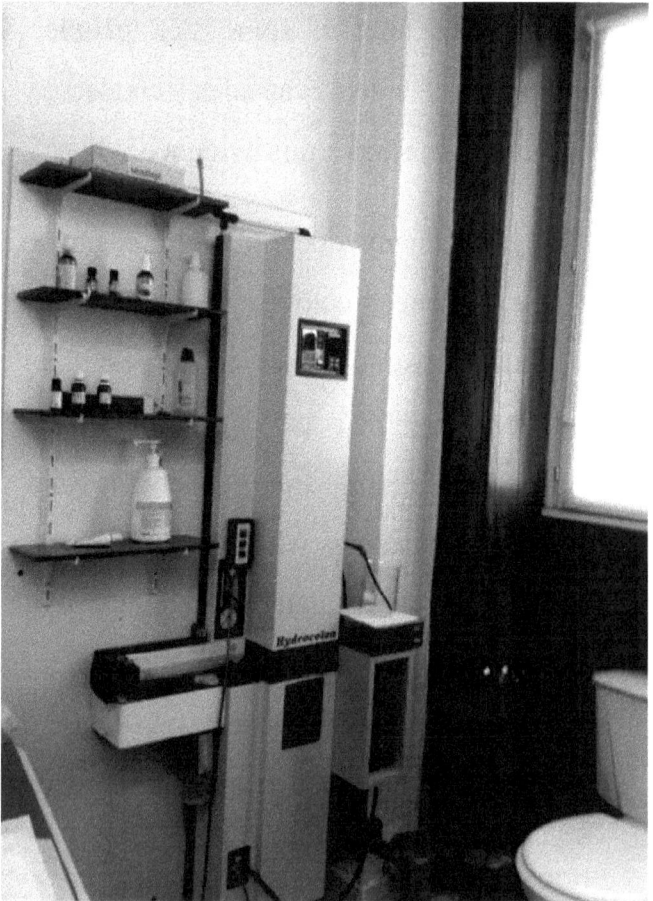

Picture of the disposable cannula and tube used with the colonic irrigation machine:

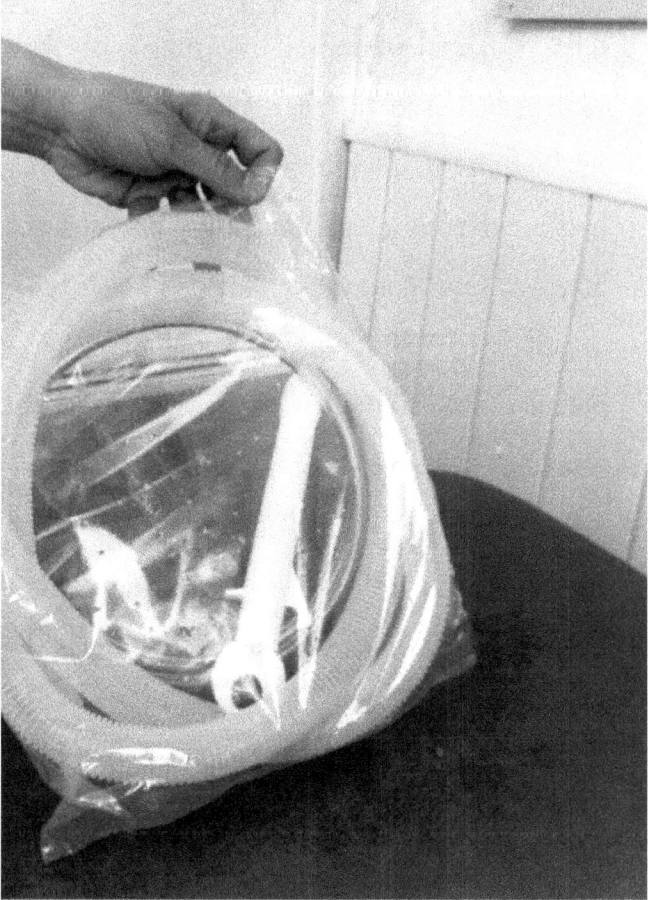

Despite all the means available to modern men and women to clean their colon, too many people still believe that a simple laxative is enough. Even worse, many believe they are perfectly clean because they go to the bathroom once a day. A friend of mine, who had a big belly on which she used to rest her elbows, assured me that thanks to a colonoscopy she knew that she had a perfectly clean and pinky colon. However, after a few colonic irrigations, her big belly disappeared. Which at first bothered her a lot, because she no longer knew where to rest her elbows! Just think for a moment: if you need toilet paper, this means some waste also stays on the intestinal walls. Over time this can form a hardened and coated crust. If nothing is done to regularly remove the recent deposits, they dry out, harden, and become a big problem for the proper functioning of the intestines and therefore the entire body.

Laxatives have been around since the dawn of time. If they were so effective in cleansing the digestive tract, who would have bothered cleaning the colon with water enemas, or by drinking large quantities of salty water while practicing certain yoga exercises?[3]

Colon cleansing practices done with available means have existed all over the world from time immemorial. In Africa, mothers used to relieve constipated babies by blowing water into their rectum. In France, the Sun King (Louis XIV) cleaned his colon with enemas. Despite his weak constitution, attributed by his doctors to weak genetic heredity, he lived almost 77 years. A very old age that many current European men don't reach today.

In seventeenth century France the famous author Molière used to make fun of doctors about their exaggerated use of enemas and bloodletting.

---

[3] https://www.kashikriyayoga.org/en/intestinal-cleansing/

Nobody would do this now because French doctors are no longer interested in these practices.

Basic techniques for disease prevention are no longer taught in modern medical schools. Indeed, from a certain age on, many doctors also have cluttered intestines and baby bumps, despite their medical knowledge and all the pharmaceutical laxatives available on the market. If ingesting laxatives were enough to stay clean inside, everybody would effortlessly live at least one hundred years in full health, in good shape, and without depending on drugs to survive. Unfortunately, reality shows that this is not the case. Many people don't live that long, and the very few who reach an "old age" do so with the help of drugs. In rich countries today the majority of people who live from 75 to 90 years old suffer from multiple pathologies due to a high level of internal dirt. It would be more logical to help them clean their bodies instead of prescribing them drugs to treat all the diseases caused by a "clogged" body.

Some doctors have claimed that autopsies often reveal the incredible cluttered state of the colon of so-called elderly people. Sometimes they find pounds of compacted waste accumulated inside the intestines from a lifetime, having left only a little free space for a poor daily bowel movement. As Hippocrates put it, "Death begins in the colon." Fortunately, by cleaning the colon, this inevitable appointment can be significantly delayed. Above all, colon cleansing can help avoid suffering for twenty or thirty years before death, spending all those years seeking treatments and visiting doctors and hospitals instead of living an active, happy, and creative life.

While cleaning the outside of the body is easy, cleaning the inside is not. It is even harder now because we ingest all kinds of unnatural products: food full of pesticides, polluted air and water, not to mention our chemical drugs. It is striking that we have become aware of the necessity of ecology in regard to the environment, but we ignore it for our body, continuing to give it polluting chemicals as medication. In my opinion, chemical drugs should be reserved for very old people who no longer have enough vitality to heal naturally, for the temporary alleviation of pain, and for difficult cases that resist a cure through natural means and better lifestyle. Every so often, the body's intelligence initiates a mandatory cleansing by triggering a disease. To avoid the occurrence of disease, which is really unpleasant and can sometimes lead to death (if there are no longer enough resources in the body to overcome the disease), we need to have a healthy lifestyle and regularly clean the inside of our body. As for women, these efforts will be amply rewarded by the total absence of menopausal symptoms, and by an even longer life expectancy compared to that of men. Just change your ideas about body and health in general, and re-evaluate some of your mental conditioning. Most of our diseases result from the gradual "pollution" of the body, which usually begins in the digestive tract. You are the master of your health; keep this power and take action. It is never too late to act and clean yourself inside. Modern medicine, despite its advances, cannot do this for you. It will only give you crutches so that you can better endure the "side effects" of all the toxins and waste you are carrying inside. No drugs will give you back your health or the radiance, which emanates from an internally and externally clean body, and even less the joy derived from living in a properly functioning body.

Scientist Alexis Carel, Nobel laureate in medicine, conducted experiments on the longevity of cells and noticed they stay alive as long as they are cleaned of their waste. In contrast, they die after a few days if they are dirty. He succeeded in keeping the heart of a chicken alive *in vitro* for about thirty years by maintaining it in a clean and nutritious liquid. Alexis Carel is credited with this sentence: "A cell that is well hydrated, well nourished, well freed from its waste will renew forever."

Obviously, our cells cannot be well hydrated, well nourished, or shed their waste when the digestive system is cluttered and clogged. Fortunately, it is almost never too late to start cleaning and getting rid of many pathologies, including so-called menopausal symptoms. The fact that so many people manage to live up to 80 years despite chronic fouling is proof of the human body's incredible resilience. If we gave the body all the respect and cares it needs, I think almost everyone could easily live to over 100 years old in good health, as long as they also keep their spirits high. A human being is not reduced to a physical body. Humans also have immaterial emotions that can impact physical and mental health, especially in case of emotional shocks and trauma.

As mentioned before, I have observed that the intestines shed their waste much better during a woman's period and that sometimes diarrhea occurs and helps further release waste. With menopause, the intestines no longer benefit from this natural cyclical impulse for better elimination of waste. Whenever diet or emotions trigger constipation, feces accumulate in the bowels and then begins hardening and hindering the natural peristaltic waves of the intestines. All that gives place to a vicious circle of discomfort and bloating. In some cases, the intense bloating compresses the veins in the belly and hinders the correct flow of blood, leading to a variety of health issues. Bloating also affects breathing. Thus, this is often how the body begins the vicious circle of intoxication, which subsequently triggers all kinds of physical ailments, persistent negative moods, and poor assimilation of vitamins and minerals due to the slowing down of metabolism. In such circumstances, skin cells are no longer nourished well and cannot get rid of their toxins; such degradation of the skin is commonly attributed to menopause and fought with hormonal therapy, Botox, moisturizers, collagen, or even with cosmetic surgery. It is also at this point that the famous "age spots" make their appearance. According to doctors, these spots are due to lumps of melanin and are triggered by sun exposure and/or hormonal changes. Dermatologists offer the following treatments: creams to reduce the formation of melanin, age spot remover creams, cryotherapy, peeling, and laser therapy. They also advise avoiding sun exposure between 11 am and 16 pm, because they believe it is conducive to the formation of age spots.

In my forties I had big and ugly age spots covering almost half of my face, and to avoid worsening them I followed the common medical advice and did not go out without a sun hat and sunblock cream on my face. One day, after a few sessions of colonic irrigations and a fast, I was pleasantly surprised to discover in the mirror that my ugly spots had disappeared. From that I concluded that sometimes "age spots" on our faces are truly due to excessive exposure to the sun; but that in most cases they are simply "shit spots." Colon cleansing had been for me the simplest and most appropriate way to eliminate them painlessly and without side effects.

Despite the "automatic body cleansing" system enjoyed by every woman of childbearing age, "body pollution" can occur long before the onset of menopause, when this system is overwhelmed by too much waste and toxins in the body. Some "menopausal symptoms" can therefore occur long before menopause in cases of unhealthy lifestyle, food allergies, or psychological problems blocking the flow of energy in the belly and disturbing digestion and elimination. Some young women are already so intoxicated that their periods, which have become more and more uncomfortable and painful, are no longer enough to clean them. Some already show in their forties, or even in their thirties, ailments similar to those generally attributed to menopause, and may also have difficulties conceiving.

Have you now guessed why all the women in my family suffered so much from "menopausal symptoms"? It is very simple: for generations our way of cooking and eating was too greasy, too salty, too sweet, too floury, and it congested our digestive tract from childhood. Furthermore, I have found that we don't have a gluten allergy or intolerance, we simply do not digest gluten. Gluten is an extremely adhesive glue that clogs our digestive tract, hindering its correct functioning.

I, too, was struck by this "heredity"! But unlike my other family members, in my forties, long before the onset of menopause, I looked for a way to clean my digestive tract and regain my shape, my figure, and beautiful skin without age spots.

Long before the age of menopause, while my intestines were clogged mainly by undigested gluten, I already suffered from the following:

- Night sweats, especially all over the upper body, from the waist up. I was also sweating from my head and neck;

- Dry eyes;

- Extremely tense and painful breasts;

- Insomnia;

- Low mood;

- Being overweight and having a baby bump;

- Hormonal disorders, which my homeopath treated with doses of homeopathic hormones;

- And many other ailments, which, had I been in my fifties, would have been automatically attributed to menopause.

Fortunately, after my first three colonic irrigations all of this disappeared. I was especially amazed by the disappearance of the ugly large "age spots" I had on my face.

Thanks to the healthier lifestyle I started in my thirties, and colonic irrigations in my forties, my body has remained clean enough not to suffer from any of the usual inconveniences wrongly attributed to menopause. All these symptoms are actually caused by gradual intoxication and clogging of the body, starting almost always in the digestive tract.

I also associate fasting with intestinal cleansing. Colonic irrigations only clean the large intestine. However, the small intestine can also become clogged over time, and fasting is a great way to cleanse the entire digestive tract and help the body shed its toxins and waste. Intestinal cleansing combined with fasting gives excellent results.

I started fasting while living in France, where there was little information circulating about it. Later on some doctors began to take an interest in fasting and recommended it to patients with severe diseases to help them better cope with their medical treatment. Later on, fasting became more popular with the general public thanks to television broadcasts showing Russian fasting clinics where patients fasted for forty days under the supervision of teams of doctors recording information on fasting and its results. There are fasting clinics in many other countries, such as Germany and Switzerland. There are now many fasting and detox centers in France. You can find most through the magazine *Bio Contact*, distributed in health food stores throughout the country and also available online. At the end of this book you will find a list of books I found very interesting and relevant.

I did not transition overnight from my "inherited" lifestyle to fasting, colonics, and a healthy lifestyle. I began to gradually improve the way I ate, and chose better quality foods that I cooked in a much healthier way. Changing our taste in food is not easy because eating is so greatly linked to emotions and our mothers' love. Often we are seeking maternal comfort through overeating or over drinking in times of crisis. Early childhood conditioning is deeply rooted. In my opinion, it is almost impossible to change all our deep-rooted eating habits, but for ninety percent of them we can move towards better choices that are more beneficial to our health. For my part, little by little I have managed to radically change the way I eat and cook, and even a good part of my tastes. However, the only food I can ingest when I start recovering from an illness is a treat my mother used to give me: vanilla pudding. Despite not being in itself good for my health, it reminds me of my mother's love and helps me heal. I have also observed that when I have a strong desire to eat this food, I know that a disease is brewing in my body, and I often avoid it by fasting and resting.

I started fasting around my thirties, first for one day each month during my periods, drinking lots of water and resting to help my body eliminate its toxins better. Fasting for a single day is better than nothing, but it is not enough to clear the small intestine and colon of dry, compacted waste lining their walls. At that time, the thought of fasting for more than one day frightened me. I was afraid that it would result in vitamin and mineral deficiencies and I was even afraid of dying from starvation. All of this stressed me a lot.

Later on, I realized that when the intestines are dirty and do not function well there is incorrect assimilation of nutrients. By cleaning them, we start to again better assimilate vitamins and minerals from food and drinks. Even if we lose some weight during the fast, we have no problem returning to normal weight afterwards, and we feel full of strength, energy, and vitality. Conversely, when the intestines are clogged, we get very little benefit from even the healthiest food and most expensive dietary supplements.

One day I finally got over all my fears; I naturally extended my fasting period up to seven days. All the colonic irrigations I had done before, the change in diet, and my previous one-day fasts had made it easier to fast for seven days. So far, however, I have never exceeded this duration. For now, it seems to be my personal natural limit to fasting in a pleasant and happy way.

There are many books, websites, and videos explaining how to practice fasting; I mention a few in the bibliography. When I started fasting I was content to listen to my body and follow my instincts. I later studied this topic in books. All the fasting specialists say that the two most important things about fasting are the way you begin and the way you end. One should not suddenly switch from an unhealthy diet to stopping eating, nor should one resume eating large amounts of food or eat junk food at the end of a fast. One must proceed slowly and gradually. In other words, one must be very careful in preparing for the fast and even more attentive to the way in which the fast is ended. Fasting in itself is not really unpleasant if you have done a bowel cleansing and a deworming before starting it. Some people fast much longer than I do, sometimes up to forty days. Often, this long duration is necessary to overcome severe pathologies. For these long fasts it is advisable to go to specialized clinics, where it is possible to be supervised by doctors.

If you have never fasted before, you can train yourself by starting with an "evening fast" or a "morning fast," which consists of not eating in the evening or in the morning, and drinking plenty of warm water and/or herbal teas. According to Dr. Arnold Ehret, practicing intermittent fasting (*i.e.,* morning or evening fasting) for a few weeks while eating only fruits and vegetables can significantly purify the entire digestive tract. I recommend reading Arnold Ehret's book *Rational Fasting*, for interesting information about successfully practicing intermittent fasting. Alternatively, you can also go on a mono-diet or drink only freshly squeezed fruit and vegetable juice for some time.

Techniques to help cleanse the body are more effective when performed after the full moon.

Fasting is advised in all spiritual traditions. The Ancients knew, long before modern science, that we have a "second brain" in the belly that interacts with the one we have in the head. In ancient civilizations, special attention was paid to the belly inside and outside. The digestive tract was regularly cleaned and massages and specific exercises were performed. The Ancients regularly resorted to fasting, resting, and methods for emptying the entire digestive tract. In ancient times, food, water, and air were not as polluted as they are today, and bread didn't contain that much gluten!

Pollution of food, water, and environment creates toxins that the body stores when it cannot eliminate them. Digestion requires a lot of energy. Obviously it is not worth spending a lot of energy on digesting foods that in turn provide very little vitality - or worse, foods that harm us due to their increasing artificiality. In any case, to eliminate toxins well you need to have enough vitality in the body. People who have eaten poorly for years and who have never put their digestive tract to rest usually don't have enough. Some people do not stop eating when they are sick, even if they are not hungry. Sometimes they do it mainly out of habit, or because they are afraid of having deficiencies, or of dying if they stop eating for a few days. Yet nature did not plan that humans would have to eat every day, three times a day, all year round, without ever stopping.

Instead, our bodies have been wonderfully designed to survive in times of food shortage or starvation. Without this ability to run out of food for some time, humanity probably could never have thrived on the planet. The same occurs regarding animals. What do your pet dogs and cats do when they feel bad? They curl up in a corner of the house, stop eating, and let you know that they don't want to be disturbed. They won't even be tempted by their favorite treat. When they have access to a garden, some animals regularly cleanse their stomachs by ingesting grass and vomiting. To do so, they use a special breathing technique and muscular movements. I tried imitating them. It works wonders for emptying the stomach. Animals have a lot to teach us about health and above all about the best way to free the intestines. For example, if you adopt the position used by your pets when they defecate, you will experience for yourself that this is the best way to empty the intestines well. Our current posture, sitting on the toilet, is completely unnatural and absolutely harmful to health because it hinders the correct emptying of the intestines. When we defecate in a squatting position, the lower part of the colon and the rectum become aligned, and all the waste present there can go out without obstacles. If you do not have a squat toilet, and if you are not flexible enough to squat on the usual toilet, you can use a small container to put on the ground and empty it later in the toilet, or buy a "toilet step" specially designed for this purpose. It will cost you about fifty dollars on the internet. Just type "toilet step" into a search engine and you will find all kinds. A children's step can also fit, for a few dollars.

In France, we usually eat three times a day, all year round, without ever stopping. And we eat too much meat. Vegetarianism is not that popular there, and unfortunately the quality of meat continually decreases. We now have quantity but not quality in regard to food. Meat is being consumed in excess everywhere, even in places like southern Italy or Greece, where traditionally people ate very little of it. In Crete, famous for its traditional healthy diet, people now eat a lot more meat than in the past. The modern Cretan diet has nothing in common with the healthy Cretan diet of the past. As a result, the bodies of the Cretans have changed a lot, and the island is sadly facing a plague of childhood obesity. Cretan people now suffer more than ever from health issues related to the consequences of the worsening of their diet and lifestyle. There, too, people wrongly believe that laxatives can advantageously replace the ancient techniques of purification of the body; that is, fasting and intestinal washing. While older Cretans continue to eat as before and thus keep fit, children prefer hamburgers and fries from local "fast food" over the tasty and healthy meals of their grandmothers. Nor should we dare to serve them the wild herbs that Cretans usually collect in the mountain and consume in spring. Even boiled, these herbs are very rich in vitamins and minerals, and are beneficial to the body. If the Cretans boil them, it is not because they do not know that cooking eliminates some vitamins and minerals, but because they know that by

71

doing so they avoid parasites. Today, parasitic diseases affect a large part of the world's population, even in sanitized countries such as France, Italy, or the United States. In rich countries, mainstream media does not inform the population about this issue. It is considered too disgusting and therefore taboo. I will talk about it anyway, because clearing the body of parasites is of prime importance to live a happy menopause. So keep reading and you will be informed. If you are too sensitive, you may skip the next chapter. Just remember that almost all of us are infected with parasites, and that some drugs, for once almost free of side effects, are very effective in getting rid of these undesirable beings. Just ask your doctor to prescribe you a dewormer. In the most difficult cases, have your stool tested by a laboratory to choose the most appropriate dewormer. You can also try a drug that you can buy at a pharmacy without a prescription.

CHAPTER 3: One of the most important things to do to avoid so-called menopausal symptoms

Despite all I did to stay healthy, at some point in my life I started suffering from bloating, mainly under the stomach, in my small intestine, which I could not fix despite all I tried. I also observed that I no longer felt that clean. My body was getting poisoned and I did not understand why. I also noticed that fasting tired me much more than before, and that I was no longer able to fast comfortably and happily. My sleep had deteriorated, and I felt quite tired without understanding why. After a short fast, instead of feeling better I was particularly weak and exhausted; my stomach was even more swollen and I suffered from water retention. I didn't understand what was happening, and why all my usual practices for cleansing my digestive tract did not stop the bloating. At this point, I decided to try a technique I learned in a course on the use of dreams to better manage health. [4] This technique is used to see the inside of the body in the dream state. It sounds extraordinary, but it is very simple. This is how I came to understand that my bloating was due to parasites in my small intestine. In her book *Your Dreams Can Save Your Health*, Anna Mancini gives some examples of frequent and common dreams that inform the dreamer there are parasites in the body.

Do you know the origin of the expression "How are you doing?" It goes back to the Middle Ages and was a medical question, equivalent to asking: "How are you going to the bathroom?" In other words, "What is the consistency, appearance, and odor of your feces?" It is by observing our feces that we can learn a lot about our state of health,

---

[4] Course conducted by Anna Mancini, who has written many original and useful books on dreams; her website: www.amancini.com.

and above all we can regularly check whether we, like our cats and dogs, harbor parasites in our digestive system.

We are accustomed to deworming our pets and sometimes our small children, but very few people think about deworming themselves regularly. I was like that too, and without the dream I had, I would never have imagined that my unusual health issues could have been caused by parasites in my small intestine. Yet humans have always defended themselves against parasites. It is only in our current time that this issue seems to have become taboo in rich countries. As a result, we have let our guard down and very little information circulates on the prevention of parasitism in humans, as well as on their necessary regular elimination. Hence, parasites have taken advantage of this situation to proliferate, and they now affect a bewildering proportion of the population. It is estimated that about eighty percent of the world's population is heavily parasitized without knowing it. If intestinal worms ate the waste accumulated in our intestines, they would do us a great service. But this is not the case, and some even behave like vampires, clinging to the intestinal walls and sucking our blood. Other parasites have settled just below the stomach, in the small intestine, where they get the best from our freshly digested food. They leave us only the remains of our food and also their ammonia-filled waste, which poisons the body, disturbs the brain, and causes insomnia. When their population is large enough, intestinal worms can also cause intestinal obstruction, and it is sometimes during a surgery that the actual cause of a patient's digestive problems is discovered by chance! It is a shame to get to this point, when modern drugs can easily free our bodies of many kinds of parasites. We must accept the idea that even as "clean adults" we can nevertheless host these creatures.

Parasites can take advantage of us for years, sometimes without being noticed by any symptoms other than gradual health decline, accelerated aging, nightmares, dark circles around the eyes, sadness, tired eyes, bad digestion, bloating, and decreased muscle mass.

People used to regularly perform deworming practices. Now this is hardly the case; yet we have never been more exposed to all kinds of parasites. We do not need to travel to pick them up; they reach us through fruits, vegetables, people, animals, plants, and all that comes to us from all over the world.

It is so easy to get parasitized that almost all of us are infected, sometimes from birth. Parasites are also transmitted through the placenta, breast milk, and by contact. Veterinarians know this, which is why they recommend deworming females at the time of mating, and every two weeks before and after they give birth. As for puppies and kittens, they recommend deworming them every fortnight until the age of two months, and regularly thereafter.

While most people have no problem accepting that their pets have parasites, they are nauseated if they are told they should also deworm themselves regularly if they want to stay healthy. Dr. Hulda Clark claimed it might be enough to be licked by a cat or dog to pick up some parasites.

The main reason humans no longer deworm themselves is medical misinformation, coupled with fear and disgust at the thought that these creatures are somehow devouring us from the inside, while also releasing their metabolic waste into our bodies. At first glance it is a real horror movie – it causes many people to ignore this problem, even if not taking action means leaving the door open to all the pathologies that can be triggered by parasites. On the internet the professionals who most actively warn against parasites are veterinarians, not doctors. Go check. By typing "dewormer" into a search engine, you will come across a wide variety of products for deworming animals, especially cats, dogs, and horses. There is far less information and choice of products for us humans.

In our current living conditions, a body free from parasites has a hard time staying clean over the years. But a parasitized body can no longer stay clean, even if colon irrigation and fasting are practiced. Parasites endure our fasting much longer than we do, and it is much more difficult to fast when we have parasites because they release substances that trigger in us a tremendous hunger and irresistible attraction toward all the sweet and junk foods they like.

A parasitized person tends to eat a lot more and thus put a strain on her digestive system without getting enough energy from the food she has ingested. As a result, she quickly loses energy and feels a sadness and fatigue that triggers her desire to consume more and more addictive substances such as coffee, tea, alcohol, sweets, and drugs. Gradually, the body becomes more and more poisoned, and lacks the necessary vitality to eliminate its toxins and those of its parasites. This is the beginning of a vicious cycle of quickly deteriorating health.

The presence of parasites in the digestive system, which often goes hand in hand with the congestion of this system, leads to more clogging and accelerated aging of the body. This in turn triggers disorders that are considered to be menopausal symptoms when they occur in women in their fifties, and disorders attributed to aging after that period.

It is easy to understand that if we do nothing to regularly eliminate intestinal parasites, the more years that pass, the more the parasites proliferate in the body. They sometimes reach a critical mass, which, together with the waste accumulated in the colon over the course of life, can sometimes lead to intestinal obstruction.

Medicine is a difficult art, and today's doctors, submitted to increasingly burdensome red tape, can no longer devote enough time to each patient. Consequently, we all should take responsibility for our own health, and bother with regular checking for the presence of parasites in our stool. Most doctors won't think about parasites when a patient consults them for digestive disorders, nervousness, or sleep disorders. I know people who have consulted all sorts of conventional or alternative doctors for years, and have taken all sorts of allopathic and natural remedies, only to find one day by chance, looking down in the toilet, that their digestive disorders and/or insomnia were simply due to the presence of worms in their digestive tract!

If you don't feel like looking at your stools, here are some symptoms that signal the presence of parasites in the digestive system:

- Insomnia, nervousness, bruxism;
- Bloating, baby bump;
-Reduction of muscle mass;
- Alternation of diarrhea and constipation;
- Anemia;
- Chronic fatigue;
- Dark circles under the eyes and a sad and tired face;
- Low mood, pessimism, depressive states;
- Appetite disorders;
- Addictions;
- Craving for sweet foods and junk food;
- Itching on the tip of the nose and / or other parts of the body;
- Ridges or white spots on the nails;
- Age spots on the face;
- Tachycardia;
- Anxiety, nightmares;
- Food intolerances and allergies.

However, some people, even heavily infected, may have no other symptoms than a gradual drop in energy and a little sadness.

I now deworm myself regularly, and I have also introduced preventive substances into my diet, such as pumpkin or papaya seeds, thyme, ginger, cinnamon, oregano, pepper, etc. I also occasionally use an allopathic dewormer. I did a garlic cure, which did me a lot of good, but had no effect on my parasites. Although garlic is said to be a powerful dewormer, it perhaps doesn't work for all types of parasites.

If you often have dark circles around your eyes, even when you sleep enough and don't drink alcohol, instead of masking them with some make-up take a mild deworming drug for a few days. The results will be extraordinary and will last longer than make-up!

I cannot recommend any medications or remedies because I am not a doctor. But I can tell you there are many types of natural herbal dewormers. I have tried many of them, but have observed that allopathic drugs are much more effective for me, and have fewer side effects than all the natural antiparasitics I have tried. Some plants are too strong for me, and they disturb my liver and bowels. Allopathy has proven to be milder and more effective than plants for me. I also tried Dr. Hulda Clark's zapper, a device that emits micro electric currents that destroy parasites. This tool is interesting, but unfortunately it cannot eliminate the parasites we host in our intestines, where they are protected from electrical discharges. Hulda Clark clearly warned in her books that her zapper could not kill the parasites located inside the intestines. Instead, she recommended an herbal blend to kill the worms and eggs located in the digestive tract. This is composed of walnut (*juglans Nigra*), wormwood, and cloves. This program is described in her book *The Cure for All Diseases*. It is easy to find the details of this anti-parasites program on the internet. Zappers can help kill parasites living outside the digestive tract and you will find many kInds of zappers on the internet, at all price points. The one I tried cost about 70 USD, and after a week of use I had a noticeable health improvement. Hulda Clark claims that most diseases are caused by the presence of parasites in the body.

I waited until the end of this book to talk about this important problem and its consequences on menopause because it is a "very sensitive" topic about which people generally don't want to hear. Neither fasting nor intestinal cleansing can rid the body of certain intestinal worms, particularly those that are firmly attached to the wall of the intestines, where, like little vampires, they are continually sucking blood. It is impossible to get rid of them with enemas when they live in the small intestine, unreachable by the water of enemas or colonic irrigations.

Obviously, to promote health, it is best to proceed in this order: start with a deep deworming, then do a colonic irrigation, then finish with a fast. Everything will be much better if you proceed in this order. If you have been parasitized for a long time, you will need to take deworming drugs several times, and then regularly resort to herbal blends and other natural remedies to avoid new infestations. This is especially true if you live in close contact with pets.

Parasites can be responsible for some "menopausal disorders," including nervousness, low mood, depression, hormonal imbalances, and insomnia. All these ailments can easily be avoided when they are simply due to parasites. When in doubt, an anti-parasite drug is worth a try. If you feel better right away, and if your "menopausal symptoms" suddenly disappear, you will know what was causing them.

Now I would like to speak about some "miracle" cures and products that are supposed to cleanse the colon quickly and effortlessly. Then I will speak about the foods that are more conducive to the clogging of our digestive tract.

CHAPTER 4: Some considerations on "miraculous remedies" to cleanse the body and foods that clog the digestive tract

Alternative "miraculous remedies."

With the trend of natural health, easy techniques to get rid of our toxins or to free the intestine from waste are promoted on the internet. Unfortunately, most only "free" our wallet and/or mislead us, letting us believe we are perfectly clean inside, while we are still full of waste. Let's speak about some of them.

Plants in capsules.

Blends of plants, sold in capsules, often reach very high prices compared to the individual loose plants they contain. Furthermore, ingesting dry plants in large quantities can also contribute to obstructing the digestive system, as they are difficult to assimilate in this form. I noticed while looking at my stools that most of the time - and especially when there are parasites in the body – these capsules simply come out undigested and are not at all accepted or used by my body. Herbal teas, decoctions, and oils of these same plants are often much better assimilated by my body. Obviously, everyone is different, and it is worth observing what comes out of your body in order to understand what you can or cannot assimilate. Plants are of great help in cleaning our digestive system, but we must choose them wisely and take them in the form that best suits our metabolism. Herbal blends that are supposed to clear the intestines of old waste are sold at high prices and are not as effective as cleansing the intestines with water and fasting. I tried many when I was in the US and most of these blends disturbed my body without actually cleaning me up. In fact, these blends are mostly made up of laxatives, which would cost a lot less at the pharmacy!

The cleaning of the liver and gallbladder with olive oil and grapefruit.

Certain liver and gallbladder cleansing practices have become popular mainly thanks to Andreas Morritz and Hulda Clark. I have tried the liver cleansing procedure several times, resulting in my health declining. It seemed really violent to my body and I found that the large number of stones released did not come from my liver, but were only "oil stones" due to the large quantity of the mixture of olive oil and grapefruit juice I had ingested, according to the recommended liver cleansing protocol advocated by these authors. However, I believe this procedure may be useful in cases of extreme emergency because, according to many testimonies, it has often avoided the surgical removal of the gallbladder. For my part, I prefer the gentler, traditional methods of draining the liver and gallbladder. I avoid being violent with my body and stressing it when there is a milder alternative. For those interested, I have listed the books of Hulda Clark and Andreas Morritz in the bibliography. To their quick violent fixes, I prefer intermittent fasting practiced for a long time, which gradually cleanses the whole body, including the liver and gallbladder, provided you learn how to do it intelligently.

Magnesium.

The ingestion of magnesium (or Epsom salts) is deemed to purify the digestive system but it acts as a laxative that evacuates only the most recent waste, but not those hardened and compacted, sometimes tightly attached for decades to the walls of the intestines. Magnesium taken orally is bad for the digestive system and is scarcely assimilated. Since most of us are deficient in magnesium, it would do us good if only it was absorbed well. The solution is to absorb it through skin, in liquid form. I regularly put "oil of magnesium" on my skin from where it is absorbed much better than in the digestive tract. You can easily find this product on the internet by typing "magnesium oil" into a search engine.

Psyllium and psyllium-based miracle formulas.

Psyllium, popular in Ayurveda (Indian medicine) is renowned for helping cleanse the digestive tract. However, it should be taken with some precautions, as it can contribute to clogging a digestive system already loaded with lots of compacted waste and parasites. Psyllium absorbs a huge amount of water when immersed. It is often incorporated into miracle products (which cost much more than just the inexpensive psyllium) that are supposed to cleanse the colon perfectly, quickly, easily, and spectacularly According to some advertisers, you can ingest just one of these "magical remedies" (made

93

mainly with psyllium) and see with your own eyes the extraordinary and tangible results. Such "results" are shown in promotional videos on the internet. Sometimes they can be shocking to sensitive people because they show huge, rubber-looking lumps that were supposedly blocked for years in the intestine. In reality these "giant lumps" are not some old intestinal deposits released thanks to these products, but simply the products themselves processed by the body. Just as other videos demonstrate, by immersing these products in a bowl of water, and leaving them for a while at temperatures close to that of the stomach, we can see the same "giant lump" forming in the bowl. Unfortunately, these products do not dissolve the dry, compacted waste matter stored in the intestine. Perhaps they help a little in dragging out the most recent deposits.

Used cleverly, psyllium, flaxseed, mild laxatives, and other plants can help the body rid itself of recently accumulated waste. They are also useful as preliminaries for colonic irrigations or enemas. However, they cannot rid the digestive system of all the waste that has accumulated, hardened, dried, and compacted for decades. Once a state of advanced congestion has been reached, it is necessary to use the means that have proven most effective: colonic irrigation sessions and fasting. As for intestinal flora, these disorders very often derive from the unsuspected presence of intestinal parasites for years. So, in such a case, taking probiotics is of little use as long as you are housing these parasites and do not take appropriate action to eliminate them.

Until now I have spoken about the ways to unblock your pipes! Now, let me explain what tends to clog them. Obviously, digestive congestion isn't just due to our foods. Emotions play an important role in digestion and intestinal movement.

According to the teachings of yoga, food passes through six valves whose proper functioning can be affected by muscular tensions and negative emotions. Furthermore, sitting during and after meals is not conducive to good digestion. This position compresses our organs and decreases our digestive and respiratory capacity and our peristalsis (rhythmic movement of the intestine). Movement during the day is recommended to improve intestinal peristalsis and thus promote good transit.

Foods conducive to clogging the intestines.

Many authors of alternative medicines claim that poorly digested foods contribute to the obstruction of our intestines. Arnold Ehret, author of a book called *The Mucus Free Diet*, recommended cutting out almost all flour-based foods, cheeses, and even legumes from our diet, and eating mainly fruits and vegetables. I tried this diet and observed that it was beneficial for digestion and bowel movement. In contrast, through observing my stools, I easily noticed that pasta, bread, pastries, cereals, cheese, white rice, biscuits, when eaten alone and once mixed with my bile, usually formed some compact and sticky masses difficult to digest and evacuate. When these foods are undigested and blended with bile, they are extremely detrimental to our health by clogging all of our digestive tract. Not to mention the undigested gluten that forms such a sticky glue that the body cannot get rid of it without our help. Yet, at the same time, these foods are those that seem to bring us so much energy. Ancient legends say that the invention of wheat, transmitted by the gods, was a great turning point for humanity because it made men stop devouring each other. Symbolically, this means that, thanks to wheat, any individual had enough energy and did not need to steal it from others. By observing my stools, I realized that it is possible to continue benefiting from gluten-free cereals in all their forms, if we eat them in small quantities and always accompanied with vegetables and fibers, and if we stay well hydrated throughout the day. As for cheese and chocolate, they are a real disaster for our "pipes" when eaten alone. A piece of goat cheese or Gruyere eaten alone forms a compact mass that is very difficult to evacuate. Again, only eat cheese in very small quantities and serve it not with bread, but with vegetables containing enough water and fiber, or with ripe fruit. If you want to eat some chocolate, eat it with fruit. Adopting the fruits and vegetables diet recommended by Ehret effectively rests and cleanses the body.

It is by observing your stools that you can understand how your body reacts to the foods you eat. You may understand from their odor after eating meat or fish that these foods are probably not suitable for you. Everyone is different, and it is by observing yourself that you can learn how to eat properly and do yourself good with the food you ingest Some people may experience diarrhea from eating the same foods that cause constipation in others. Trendy diets and dietary fads advocated by medical or naturopathic authorities have always existed. It is only by observing your bowel movements that you will be able to figure out which diet is the most appropriate for you and which foods you should avoid. You will also notice that this diet varies according to the season and location.

Foods that contribute to the creation of excess mucous in the body.

Many alternative medicine authors have denounced the harmful effects of milk and dairy products. They claim they turn into mucus, building up in the body and preventing its proper functioning.

I have never been much attracted to dairy products and have not developed a habit of consuming them much. After reading books and articles warning about the adverse effect of eating dairy, I decided to make the following experiment. I only ate three natural yogurts a day for three days, and I repeated this experiment several times. As a result, I noticed that these dairy foods created an incredible amount of mucus in my intestines. I then decided to cut dairy from my regular diet. I also realized that I did not eat them because I loved them, but only because I had been conditioned by school and television to consider them as healthy foods and an almost irreplaceable source of calcium. In the 1960s all French schools had a morning break during which all the children lined up to receive a glass of milk. What a good deal for the country's dairy industries, which had taken advantage of this to advertise even more and develop their range of dairy products, full of harmful additives.

I still remember very well the song from the advertisement: "Dairy products are our friends for life ... la la .... Dairy products, for life." But I no longer believe in this, because I have observed for myself that they are quite the opposite. As far as I am concerned, milk causes diarrhea and yogurt forms mucus in my body. Dairy products are no longer part of my usual diet, but I still eat them occasionally whenever I greatly desire them. I believe that it is important not to feel deprived. Sometimes we are strongly attracted to some foods considered "unhealthy" because our body badly needs something it contains.

By gradually adopting a healthier lifestyle, our tastes change and we no longer feel deprived of the junk foods we used to enjoy because we no longer like them.

Eating something bad for our health from time to time, but that makes us happy, isn't necessarily bad in the end. It gives our body the opportunity to train its elimination systems. Generally, our bodies have no problem eliminating small amounts of occasionally ingested "poisons." However, large quantities repeatedly ingested over a long time is another story that alone causes, in my opinion, 95% of so-called menopausal symptoms, while the remaining 5% is mainly due to our mind, which in some cases hinders the correct flow of energy in the body. Our intestines also produce hormones and they can trigger hormonal disturbances when they are not functioning well.

To conclude this book on an optimistic note, I now want to tell you what menopause should be and what positive changes it should normally bring to every woman.

CONCLUSION

Experiencing menopause in physical and mental well-being, that is, in full health, is in itself admirable, but there are also some good surprises that await women who have taken care of their bodies and have been strong and intelligent enough to avoid all the traps of mainstream media propaganda about menopausal women and its disastrous image. Such image has never been more negative than today. Eva Lavie's poem, which I include with her permission at the end of this conclusion, is a good summary of the present situation. The way mainstream media pictures menopausal women goes hand in hand with present materialistic views of the world, in which women tend to be considered without love and as disposable sexual objects.

But the world has not always been predominantly patriarchal and materialistic. Archaeological evidence reminds us that planet Earth was once inhabited by many matriarchal civilizations. And we still have a few.

So, what happened to women? Who, in a remote past, seemed to have dominated the world, but fell to such an inferior position? Legends claim that in ancient times women had powerful psychic powers, but misused them to dominate and enslave men, to the point that they ended up losing all their powers. Once deprived of them, they fell under the physical domination of men. These are legends, but some vestiges of these ancient powers still show up through tales with female characters such as fairies and witches. If Woman has been regarded as Man's guide in many archaic societies, it is because Woman is known to be more gifted in developing psychic powers, and menopause has something to do with these gifts.

Menopause offers women the opportunity to activate their higher psychic centers with their sexual energy, rather than keeping it in the lower part of their body. The activation of these centers makes many incredible things possible. For example, it becomes easier to materialize dreams and thoughts, and to develop intuition, hypnotic ability, telepathy, clairvoyance, and, of course, healing powers.

A well-prepared and lived menopause can lead every woman to a new lease on life, much more interesting and joyful than the "destiny" our patriarchal and materialistic world seeks to impose on them. I strongly believe that a better future for humanity, animals, and the environment depends on the balance between male and female forces in our world. The main problem of our civilization is its lack of feminine values, the ones that put transmission and maintenance of life at the forefront and value life and love more than anything else.

If you liked this book, please leave a comment on the site where you purchased it. This will make it easier for other women to find. You will also help contribute to changing the image of women in menopause.

I wish you all the best and a wonderfully magical menopause. And don't forget to pay attention to your dreams during that time, you may have good surprises!

Laure Goldbright

THE ABANDONED TEMPLE

(Poem by Eva Lavie, from her book entitled: *Poésie de la vie*, published by Buenos Books International, Paris)

I am the woman of your images

Of your obscene media

And of your mirages.

I am fake from head to toe

And my soul has run away

My silicone breasts,

They no longer feed

My uterus is cold

Like the lair of death.

I'm only concerned by my appearance.

And my heart beats to the rhythm

Of your money printing machines.

Finished its cosmic rhythm!

I am the trapped woman

Of your images and your thoughts

Which have sterilized me.

My empty and depressing gaze

My smile so cold and too white

My silicone curves

Men, how these lures

Can attract you?

More than life, more than love?

More than nature?

That is abandoning me and you.

INTERESTING BOOKS FOR YOUR HEALTH

Colon Health, The key to a vibrant life!, Dr Norman W. Walker's

Home Medicine Guide, Edgar Cayce

The New Science of Healing, Louis Khune

Your Dreams Can Save Your Health: Signs of Infectious Diseases in Dreams, Dreaming the Right Remedies, Accurate Diagnosis, and Early Detection of Diseases, Anna Mancini

Depression and How Your Dreams Can Help You Avoid It, Anna Mancini

Colon Cleansing and Its Benefits for Health and Skin: A Testimonial, Laure Goldbright

The Meaning of Dreams, Anna Mancini

Tricks to Sleep Better, Anna Mancini

The Cure For All Diseases, Hulda Clark

The Liver and Gallbladder Miracle Cleanse, Andreas Moritz

www.myperfectcolon.com/ (Site presenting the intestinal cleansing device at home, with online sale of the product and accessories)

BOOKS BY LAURE GOLDBRIGHT

http://lauregoldbright.buenosbooks.fr

Colon Cleansing and Its Benefits for Health and Skin: A Testimonial

Vegetarian and Organic Paris (out of stock)

Gare à Vous les Virus !

Les Parisiens au Boulot, LOL !

10 Ans d'Études, 20 Ans de Chômage, C'est Ça la Vraie France

Bienvenue à Tous Au Concours Du Centre National de la Recherche Scientifique

CONTENTS

www.ingramcontent.com/pod-product-compliance
Lightning Source LLC
Chambersburg PA
CBHW072238290326
41934CB00008BB/1329